BDSM

for Beginners

BDSM for the Family Bedroom

purposes only. All effort has been executed to present accurate, up to date, reliable, complete information. No warranties of any kind are declared or implied. Readers acknowledge that the author is not engaged in the rendering of legal, financial, medical or professional advice. The content within this book has been derived from various sources. Please consult a licensed professional before attempting any techniques outlined in this book.

By reading this document, the reader agrees that under no circumstances is the author responsible for any losses, direct or indirect, that are incurred as a result of the use of the information contained within this document, including, but not limited to, errors, omissions, or inaccuracies.

Table of Contents

Introduction

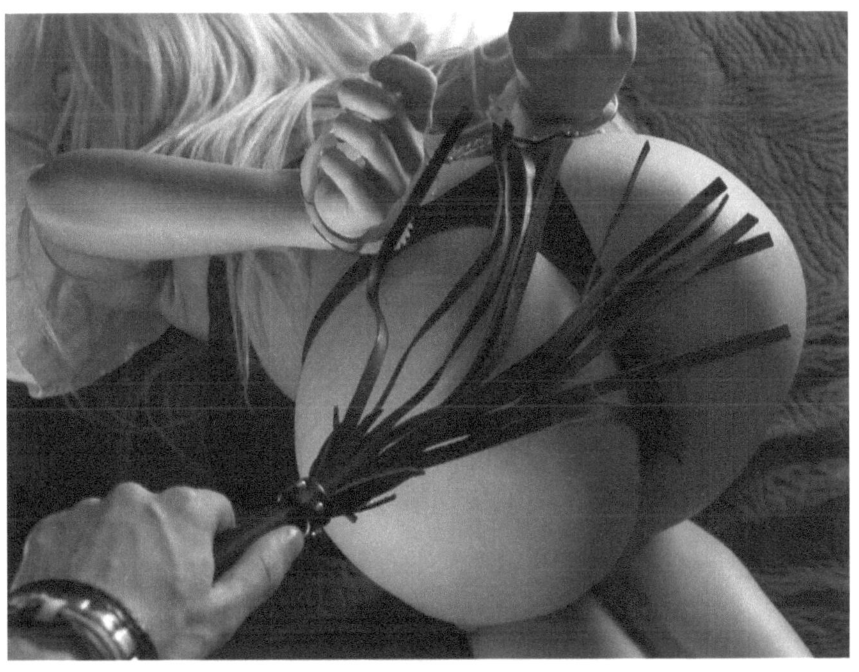

Most people are inclined to think of BDSM as a taboo, sexual deviance left for those who have a taste for latex, leather, with no limits, secrets, and a soundproof room in their basement draped in velvet and silk. The porn industry, popular novels, movies, and lyrics of some chart-topping songs can skew the overall idea a person has regarding BDSM.

Simply put, BDSM stands for bondage and discipline, dominance and submission, sadism and masochism.

BDSM, perhaps what is considered the *"harder,"* *"scarier"* stuff might turn people off completely. Yet, BDSM does not have to be about chains and whips; it can also include innocent light caresses with a feather and nothing more.

Kinky or erotic play can take place during foreplay and not during sex, or it can be included both in foreplay and sexual intercourse. It can include one element or several; you are the master of your sexual preferences, demands, kinks and fetishes.

To understand BDSM is also to understand that we are all human and in saying so are all unique, at that extends to the bedroom, what we like and do not like there. It is also important to understand that it is okay to enjoy certain things that you might think others shall think of as weird or distorted. Sex is both liberating, fulfilling, and deeply personal experience. These feelings and emotions are even more heightened when sharing it with someone whom you share a mutual respect with, such as your partner.

There is no condoning *"vanilla"* sex that leaves both participants feeling satisfied, nor is there room to scoff at what an added few spanks and, or hair tugging can add to sexual gratification. After all, your relationship might even improve with a few nights of added BDSM play.

This modern subculture has allowed many to explore their impulsiveness positively and make the bedroom a place of excitement and, most importantly, trust.

History of BDSM

It all started with whips. Whips have been a part of the world's history for eons and used throughout cultures and many religions as part of punishment, worship, and pleasure.

During earlier Roman times, women would whip each other when worshipping the god of fertility, agriculture, and wine, Bacchus.

The young men of Sparta would compete at the shrine of Artemis Orthia. She was the goddess of childbirth, fertility, hunting, and nature. The men would be whipped until one became the victor, never tiring and enduring the most lashings for the longest time, he was held in the highest regard.

In the 18th century, whipping was also one of the sexual experiences offered in brothels throughout England.

The Kama Sutra, an ancient Indian text on sexuality, goes on to explain that slapping is a passionate way to increase sexual desire, want, or yearning. The text even explains that there are special locations to slap a person, a total of six, and four methods in which to do so. The texts also elaborate on biting, teasing with the tongue, teeth, and lips, which are also ways to excite and tempt.

In centuries passed, common literature was focused on men going beyond their means for the love of their life, often a woman who is married to someone of a higher class than themselves. This pain and need inspired many books, and it is suggested that these passions and denials led to such erotic behavior.

The "S" in BDSM is for sadism, meaning deriving sexual pleasure from pain. This term was coined after a French nobleman, Marquis de Sade, whose books, most of which described intrusive sexual acts. Novels such as Fanny Hill by John Cleland and Venus in Furs by Leopold von Sacher-Masoch all contain and highlight erotic behavior deemed taboo for its time.

In the last 100 years, eroticism and kink have become more acceptable. Sex toys and costumes began to appear in the mid-1920s as ways to enhance sexual pleasure in the bedroom. By the 50s, pin-ups were common, and the rise of leather fashion and more blatant homosexuality only fuelled the interest in sex and how to increase pleasure.

Thanks to the internet, all of the above culminated and has given rise to BDSM culture and the interest in discovering more ways to add variety to the bedroom. With many online platforms, such as chat rooms, forums, online stores, and social media, the ability to explore and share are limitless.

Chapter 1: What is BDSM

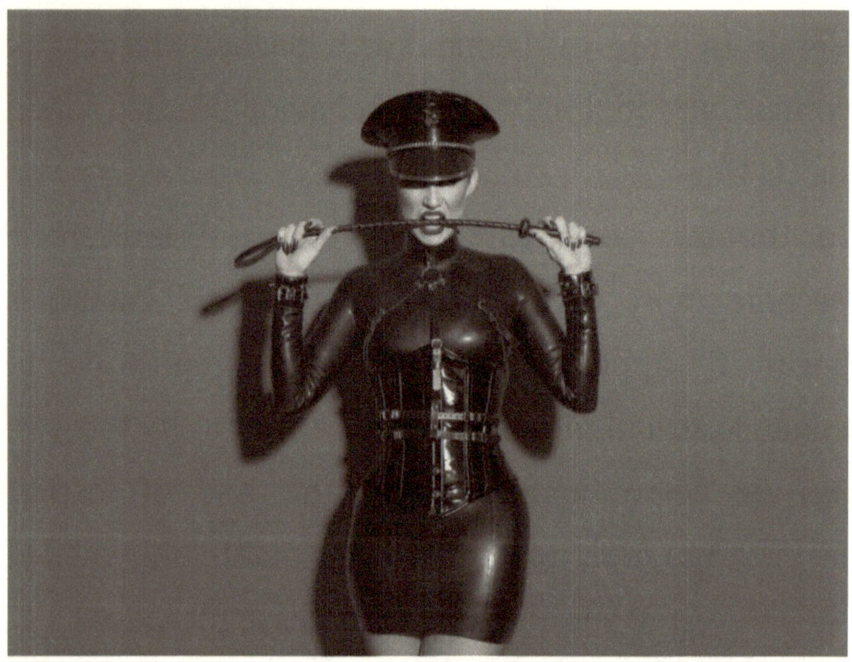

One of the most important things to remember when discussing BDSM and play is that it is always about consent.

As BDSM covers many sexual practices, most people do not align themselves entirely with this subculture. Participants might only indulge in light spanking and not much else, whereas others might choose to perform far more complex acts of bondage, sadism, and masochism nightly. The term BDSM first came into play in 1991 and welcomed all those who might have a more kinky streak inside them waiting for a chance to come out. The subculture is so far-reaching it includes cross-dressing, leather and rubber fetishes, roleplayers, and more. As mentioned, BDSM is about the equal relationship between partners, one choosing to take on a more submissive role and the other wanting to be more dominant in regards to sex and practice. BDSM may include or not include actual physical penetration; it is a question of preferences.

It is not uncommon to hear the words: *"Dom,"* *"sub,"* *"top"* or *"bottom."* These terms are frequented by those who participate in BDSM. A *"dom"* is described as the individual who takes control of the person, not only physically but psychologically. The *"sub"* is the person who is under their control. The term *"top"* is about the dominant and who controls the situation, whereas the *"bottom"* is the individual who receives the acts. A *"switch"* is whereby roles are reversed.

As of the 80s, the sexual subculture has taken on the motto: "safe, sane and consensual." Meaning that all practices are done safely, partners are both of sane mind to participate in sexual acts and both parties consent. Legally this makes BDSM ethical and above the law, especially when considering abuse and sexual assault. A partner may at any time during BDSM withdraw their consent, and you might agree on what is known as a *"safe word."* This is a word that both parties agree to use if they feel uncomfortable at any point during play and to halt it.

Initially, BDSM involves the following practices but are not limited to:

• Sadomasochism

This refers to the person either giving or receiving pain for their pleasure or sexual gratification.

- **Bondage**

Bondage refers to tying up a partner using a variety of methods, such as scarves, ropes, cuffs, or bondage tape.

- **Discipline**

Rules and role-playing are commonplace in BDSM practice. If a submissive breaks the rules, then the dominant is allowed to use forms of discipline such as spanking.

- **Dominance and Submission**

This refers to a set of rules and practices that each person undertakes for their own and partner's pleasure.

- **Female Dominance**

This is whereby the female takes on the role of the dominant partner, often termed a *"dominatrix."*

- **Female Submission**

Female submission is when a female submits to the requests, needs, and wants of their sexual partner. Generally, a partner will be of the opposite sex but can be a female dominant too. There may also be one submissive and many dominants in this form of play.

- ## Male Dominance

Male dominance is a reference to when the BDSM partner is the dominant and also a male or *"maledom."*

- ## Male Submission

In BDSM, the *"malesub"* is a male who is submissive towards a female, *"dom,"* *"domme,"* or *"dominatrix."*

The above is in no way made to put a person off but instead allow them to understand the various ways in which BDSM is conducted. Those who partake in BDSM do so consensually and, of course, at their own time and within their limits.

- ## Fantasy and Role-Playing

A fantasy can be sharing sexual secrets and wants with a partner in bed to dressing up in costumes and imagining scenarios.

- ## Fetishes

A fetish is handling a non-sexual part of the body or a non-sexual instrument in a sexual manner. Think of foot or hand fetishes or the likes of men wearing women's underwear or the love for leather, lace, or shoes.

- **Group Sex**

This includes orgies, threesomes, or sex and or swinger parties.

- **Exhibitionism and Voyeurism**

Exhibitionism can be having sex in a public space with the threat of being caught. Whereas voyeurism can include the fantasy of watching somebody engage in sexual acts without them knowing that they are being watched.

Chapter 2: How BDSM Can Improve Your Sex Life

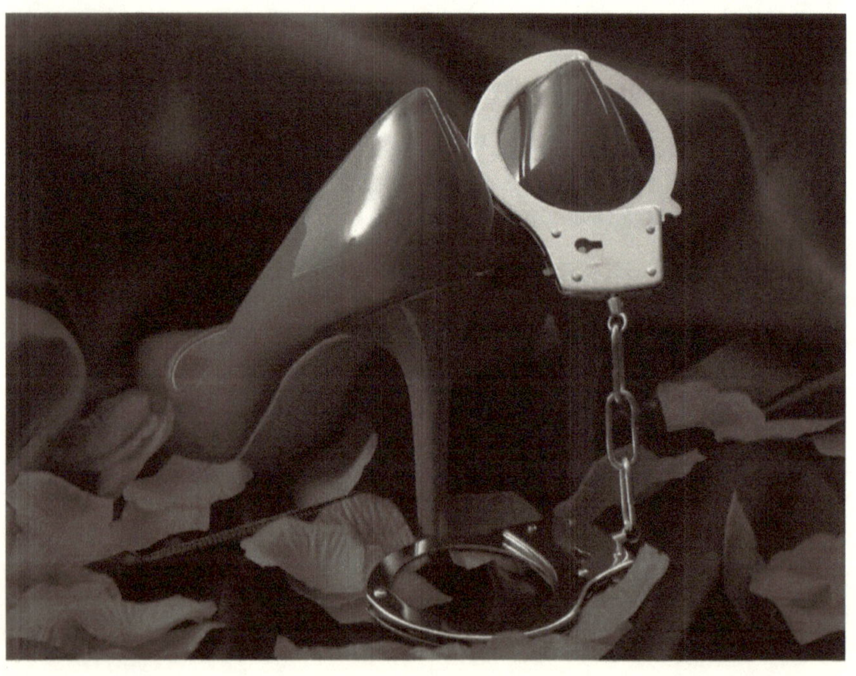

Fun fact, exhibiting more kinky behavior can improve your overall mental health and will stimulate physical health. As humans, we have an innate need for danger, and adventure, so why not in the bedroom too? Here are a few ways in which BDSM can benefit your sex life:

Boosts Your Relationship

It has been mentioned that for those who partake in BDSM, there is a remarkable emotional connection made between partners and boosts intimacy. Whips and chains might not be for you, but exchanging dirty words and light nibbling all do the same when making a very personal connection with your partner. Trust is an important facet in any relationship, and when at your most vulnerable, it is even more meaningful.

Any couple who partakes in doing various things together, such as dining out, watching a movie, or traveling, to name a few, are known to reiterate those bonds. It also alters the chemicals in your brain, and the body is rushed with dopamine, the feel-good hormone. These changes within the brain take place in the initial stages of relationships and when in-love.

Ups Mental Health

Research has suggested that there is absolutely nothing mentally or physically wrong with those who participate in any form of BDSM or fetish behaviors and are in fact considered more reasonable and balanced in all areas of their life.

Being able to express one's needs, wants, and desires without judgment and being with someone willing to participant in these acts is liberating. It also leads to the long-term joy within yourself and long-term health of the relationship.

Say Goodbye to Stress

A study conducted by members of the Northern Illinois University made mention that when partaking in BDSM activities, a person reached a mental and physical level, much like those who partake in yoga and meditation. This means that stress levels are immediately lowered. This mental state is termed *"flow"* for those who find themselves in the dominant role and *"subspace"* for those in the submissive role.

These states are said to be, apart from a gratifying experience, an enlightening one too! Why would you not want to participate in some impulsive play in the bedroom if this is what it can do for you and your relationship?

Hello to Good Health

Sex lowers your blood pressure, helps women strengthen their pelvic muscles, which help in age, more sex also makes for a stronger immune system.

Character Building

A little BDSM play can help those who are shy to become more extroverted based on the acceptance they have in the bedroom and with their partner. BDSM can help those to also be more accepting of new experiences outside of the bedroom and can help to lessen overthinking and deal with rejection better in all areas of their life. It can also provide those with confidence regarding their competency in the bedroom.

Fuels Your Libido

More sex means a greater sexual appetite. Sex changes our bodies for the better, especially in women. Due to the fact the sex releases feel-good hormones, it leaves the person yearning for more.

Common Myths About BDSM Debunked

Our opinions have certainly changed towards sexuality and sexual activities. Many mainstream movies and novels have made it more acceptable. However, they have also manipulated those into believing that BDSM is about pain and torture and a gnerally reckless endeavor.

Did you know that before 2013 and the release of the Diagnostic and Statistical Manual of Mental Disorders that BDSM play such as sadomasochism and a taste for certain fetishes was deemed to be a mental disorder by professionals in the medical arena? Research has suggested that no negative impact on the body can be found at this time about BDSM, therefore making it an acceptable practice.

Here are some common myths about BDSM and the reality:

1. You can't always tell someone is part of this lifestyle solely based on what they wear. In fact, those who participate in acts of BDSM look like your average person. Those who choose to align themselves heartfully to the movement might wear a small lock or collar as a simple gesture.

2. People who participate in BDSM are not mentally impaired or dangerous.

3. BDSM is not abuse and is a consensual agreement between partners. Those who

partake in BDSM practice take hurting an individual as irresponsible, and safety is of high importance in all regards.

4. You do not need to have a secret room for BDSM activities, nor do you need the elaborate equipment often seen in videos portraying BDSM practice. A good old wooden spoon, scarf or clothing peg, will do the trick. If you would like to venture deeper into BDSM culture and its acts, most items can be purchased at the local hardware store such as rope, rings, and chains.

5. BDSM is not about chains and whips; it is about any fetish or kink a person might have and their sexual likes and dislikes. Some choose only to dabble in light play, whereas others dedicate themselves to mastering acts of BDSM.

6. Just because an individual is dominant in their public life does not mean that they are

dominant in the bedroom. Many people often change these roles in the bedroom.

7. BDSM is both for women and men to partake.

8. BDSM is for the pleasure of both the dominant and submissive and not either-or.

Chapter 3: How to Get Started

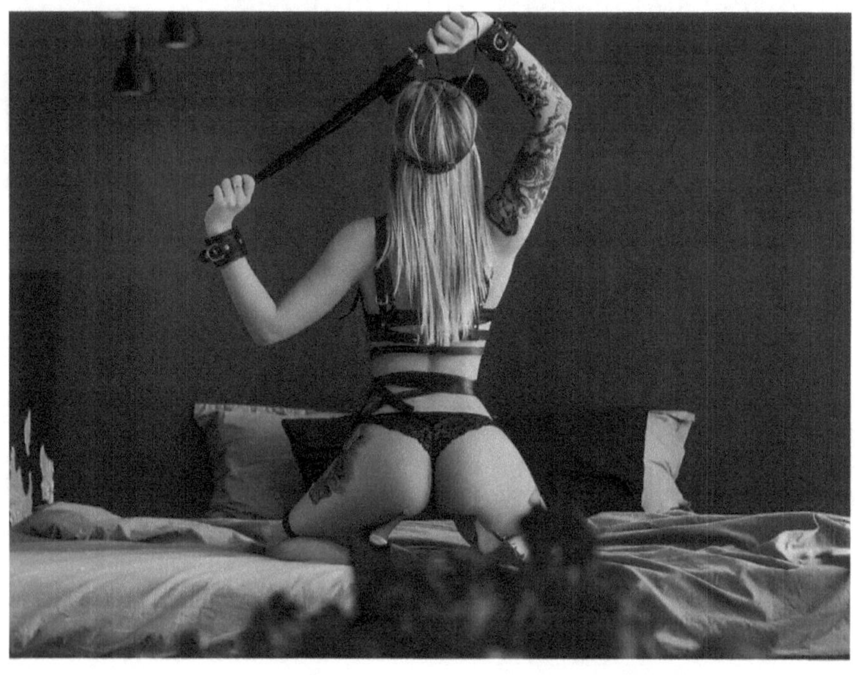

Not all aspects of BDSM have to appeal to you. However, if a few elements heighten your interest, then it would be wise to lean into these fantasies and explore them with your partner. When we imagine things, even that of a sexual nature, it provides a way of escape, and that is what BDSM partially does

Escapism from the nine-to-five workweek and other key responsibilities like raising a family.

There is no shame in wanting to explore your sexual life more broadly; it's natural. Other reasons can include the need to learn something new with your partner on a more intimate level, exchange roles of power, or to improve sex with erotic games and sex toys.

What you should understand is that getting spanked or playfully hit in the bedroom or wherever you might find yourself in a sexual encounter and aroused is the complete opposite of your partner slapping you during an argument.

A little experimentation can go a long way in confidence and pleasure.

Introducing BDSM in the Bedroom

If you know your partner well enough to talk about everything under the Sun, then you should not feel embarrassed to embark on a discussion about BDSM activities. Though initially, one can understand the hesitation.

It is advised that you broach the subject, noting specifics such as wanting to be tied up or spanked. Do not undertake to have this conversation while mid-sex. Both of you are required to be on the same page when it comes to sexual activity for it to be a pleasing experience. Discuss expectations, worries, needs, wants, likes, and dislikes. Talk about how you like to be touched or kissed in a certain manner and also encourage your partner to share the same details with you. Most importantly, never force your loved one into something that they do not want to do, you will hamper the trust that you have already built between the two of you.

A good time to mention wanting to start using a sex toy, implementing bondage, spanking, upping the dirty talk, or more regular hair pulling is when you and your partner aroused, we tend to be less likely to say no when the labido is active. Discuss BDSM over a glass of wine or in a casual environment, and always be sure to act on it soberly (at first).

Baby steps are best, start with a light spank or hair tug during sex before you whip out the cat o' nine tails. Try a sexy outfit on or even don a pair of heels. Also, try some light bondage or take turns blindfolding each other before you try all of it at once. The key is to remember is to start slow and build up momentum over time.

More importantly, know your limits, and those of your partner. There is no room for overconfidence, as you may hurt your partner or yourself. By going step-for-step can help you to act on your impulsiveness more and also assure a hesitant partner.

Are You a Switch, Submissive, or Dominant?

There is no wrong or right way when introducing BDSM practices into your relationship, nor is there a right or wrong way to conduct yourself when taking on the role of the submissive, dominant, or switch.

The best advice anyone can give you is to do only what you are absolutely comfortable with. The same way you can't expect your partner to take on a role that they do not feel is right.

The Switch Role

Many people relate more to being in a specific role than swapping between the two. Though some may choose to blur the lines, for example, you might be a dominant but have a hint of sadistic tendencies or like being a submissive but don't love the feeling of pain. Those that can swap depending on the mood, as mentioned, are called switches. The interesting part of a role as a switch is you can revel in the feelings and experiences both roles provide.

The Submissive Role

For those who take on the role of the submissive, they willingly undertake to conform to what the dominant asks of them. Dominant partners might seek for submissives to ask for their approval before touching them in a specific manner or moving in a certain way. Do not think that the pleasure is only for the dominant, being a submissive has its pros, like waiting, highly aroused, to see or feel what they will do next to you.

A submissive is generally the individual who is restrained and blindfolded. Ask your partner if they feel comfortable being called *"sir"* or *"master"* in order to delve deeper into the role of the submissive. You will also be the individual who is spanked or flogged, depending on your limits. You might also want to ask your partner if you may do certain things, such as: "S*ir, may I orgasm?"*

A few roles to get you into the mood of the submissive can be:

- Doctor and nurse (or patient)
- Headmaster and student.
- Master and servant
- CEO and secretary
- Kidnapper and victim
- Jailer and prisoner

To add even more kinky to your relationship, you might choose to play the role of submissive in public, walking behind them, acting in a specific manner, or following their commands. It is invigorating to give up your control and to place your trust in somebody else.

How to be a good submissive:

- Communicate with your dom about what they did well and what they can improve on; the idea is to be candid with each other.
- All people make mistakes, be patient with your dominatrix or dom.
- Find out the best way to please them.
- Serve them and obey their orders.
- Always use the safe word when you feel uncomfortable.
- Be physically, mentally, and emotionally present when engaging in any BDSM activities.
- During negotiations regarding our limits, be sure to mention anything that bothers you and what you do not like.
- Understand what trust and abuse are.

- Don't allow yourself to be pressured into trying anything that you are not game for.

The Dominant Role

With regard to taking on a dominant role, men might choose to align themselves more than women, but as mentioned, there is no correct or incorrect way to go about your role. Sometimes it is easier to take on a title of power, such as *"mistress," "queen,"* or *"king"* and *"ruler."*

Why not try wearing clothes and fun accessories to establish your role as the dominant, such as a pair of high heels or a chain.

It's important to remember that as a dominant, you take on the overall responsibility of a submissive, as well as respect and care for them. Knowing your partner's limits and, of course, not pushing or placing them into situations which they don't agree. As a dominant, you will be wielding most of the equipment, such as ropes, belts, and various sex toys. Try these out before you use them on a submissive, this will also allow you to gauge your strength and stamina. Remember: When you find yourself in the dominant role, the aim is to start slow and soft, building up momentum with the consent of the submissive and within their limits.

Tips on being a good dom:

- Keep your and submissive's safety a top priority.
- Know the difference between play and abuse.
- Respect your submissive's likes and dislikes.
- You can be a loving dominant versus a cruel one.
- Always keep the line of communication open.
- Stop when the sub uses a safeword.

Chapter 4: How to Practice BDSM Safely

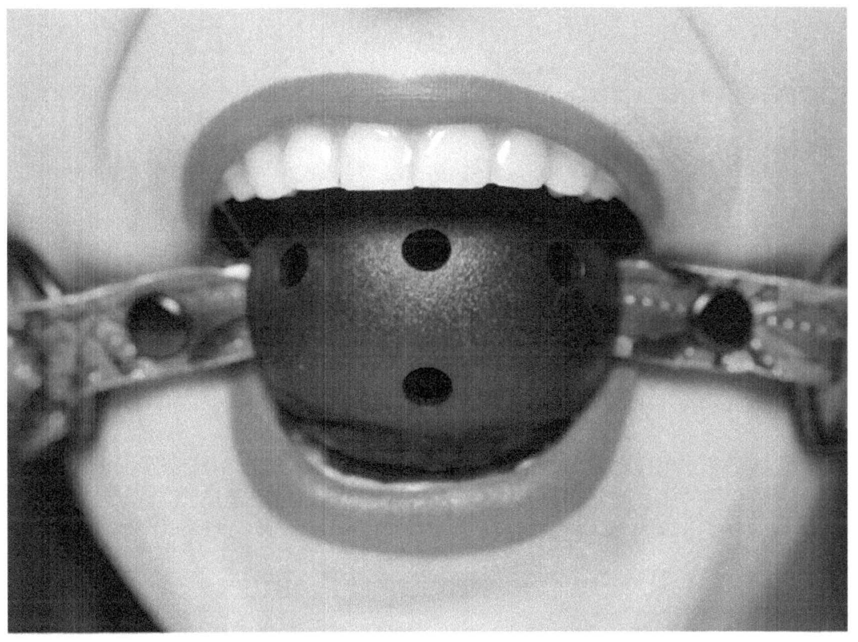

Any BDSM practices should be undertaken safely and consensually. Many align themselves with the SSC ideology, as previously mentioned: *"safe, sane and consensual."* Another ideology worth mentioning is RACK: *"risk-aware consensual kink."*

A "*scene*" is also a BDSM term in reference to a pre-planned location where acts of BDSM are conducted. There is always a beginning and an end to scenes. Talking through this beforehand is a great way of knowing what to expect when you are a bit more involved in BDSM practices. It also allows for downtime afterward as scenes can be both emotionally and physically taxing on both individuals.

Some acts, such as playful spanking might occur naturally during a normal sexual encounter and in the heat of the moment, which is fine too. Always discuss each other's limits. A person who finds themselves in a dominant position will know what their partner's hard limits are and, respectively, not push the individual further. Hard limits are things that you will never want to try, and what you are willing to try is known as soft limits. Both of which, once again, need to be established with your partner. Scenes do not need to be a serious discussion as if it's a legal proceeding but can be a casual conversation, such as: "I do not like when my feet are tied." Set up a self-created survey for you both to tick off depending on your sexual preferences. The internet is a useful tool to delve deeper into sex, toys, acts, and practices. This checklist will only strengthen your understanding of what your partner is into and against.

Contracts might seem more suited to those who partake in more edgier acts of BDSM but might clear the air when it comes to what you are comfortable doing and not doing. The contract might go on to further include the names you call each other and also make mention of a safe word.

Keep safe words short and use something easy to remember. Do not use the words "no" or "yes" as these might occur during a scene, which includes role-playing — try a three-color system, much like a traffic light. Green is go, orange means slow down, and red stops the whole thing.

It is also important to note the following with regards to BDSM and practicing safely:

- Keep a pair of scissors nearby in case you cannot untie restraints.

- Always keep the key to locks nearby.
- Keep the number of the hospital, ambulance, or paramedic on hand in case of emergencies, no matter how trivial.
- Sterilize all sex toys and items used, such as paddles before and after use.
- Silk scarves can cut off circulation; it would be wise to consider another fabric.
- A collar is ok, but do not tie something around your partner's neck as you might run the risk of asphyxiating them.
- Treat all open wounds if any occur immediately after the scene.
- Regularly check and keep your medical kit stocked.
- If you would like to experiment with spanking or making use of a cane, paddle, or whip, it is important to know not to strike a person on their lower back. You run the risk of damaging vital organs such as the liver and kidneys. Stick to the buttocks and back of the thigh, they are best because that's where the extra padding is.

Any sexual encounter causes a release of hormones, but the hormones released are far more during acts of BDSM. It is important to remember that irrespective of the intensity of your BDSM practices something called "*sub drop*" can occur. This is when hormones and chemicals begin to settle down, and feelings of guilt, pain, or crying can be experienced.

To stave off sub drop "*aftercare*" is a key element when a scene has ended. Aftercare is anything that allows those involved to resurface and rejoin the world slowly. Cuddling, eating, and drinking and staying warm are elements of aftercare that should always be implemented and help the body and mind balance themselves out again. Communication is key in any relationship and is one of the foundation blocks of BDSM.

Lastly, remember to keep all sex toys, bondage items, and any extras locked in a box and placed in a cupboard to keep them private and sterile.

Chapter 5: Sexual Pleasure Points

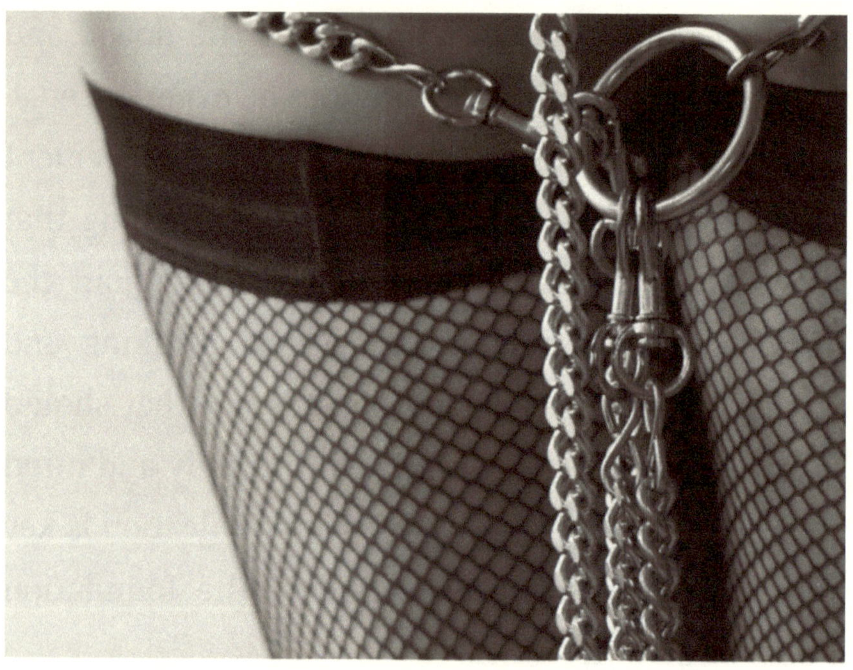

The human body has a network of nerves that travel from the top of our heads down to our toes. Many areas of the body can be stimulated to intense desire and sexual need.

Our first fumbles during sex prepare us for many years of discovering our bodies and those of others.

It also helps us learn what we enjoy and what we do not. Perhaps there is a preference for a specific position, or there is a distaste for a certain sexual act.

Many people think that the genitalia is our only vessel for immense pleasure, but as you will begin to understand, there is so much more and plenty of other places that can be massaged, touched, stroked, or pinched to guide you in the direction of ultimate pleasure. BDSM allows those who participate to explore the areas of the body and to chart their very unique pleasure points with a partner who is there to follow instructions. Here are some pleasure points you did not think you have:

Mental Connectivity

Women and men alike love to connect on a deeper, and meaningful level. These feelings create lust, want, and yearning. Perfect for igniting the flame and keeping it alive in the bedroom.

Below the Belly Button

Try stroking or tickling your partner below the belly button or just above the pubic bone. The sensations felt here are of intense anticipation. In women, the vaginal muscles contract, which may lead to orgasm alone, and for men, it is the same.

Head

When the head is massaged, our bodies release oxytocin, the feel-good hormone. This hormone, apart from soothing us, can cause sexual arousal. Start your bedroom routine off with one of these before bringing out the naughtier stuff.

Neck and Ear Lobes

The nape of the neck is an erogenous zone. When delivering a head massage, remember to pay attention to this area too. Kisses or any other form of stimuli to this area will cause toe-curling sensations. Be sure to add a nibble to the ear lobes or place the ear lobe between your thumb and index finger and gently pull downwards, it works!

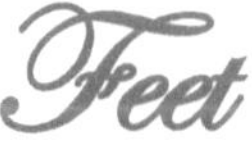

Feet

Tease or apply pressure to the soles of men and tickle or pinch the toes of women.

For men, applying pressure to the center soles of their feet is considered an important acupuncture point called the *"bubbling spring."* Applying pressure to this area relieves stress, and these sensations travel, like a bubbling spring, upwards past the genitalia.

With regards to women, soft tickling or toe sucking is just as effective, if tempted, give her big toe a steady pinch, holding it between your fingers. If you can do this while she orgasms even better.

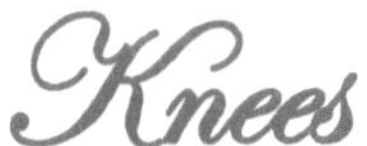

Knees

Specifically, the back part of the knee is a sensitive spot when undertaking a bit of BDSM play. Kissing them softly or giving them a light swat deliver the same sensation.

Lower Back

The small of a woman's back is highly sensitive to touch. Remember to pay attention to that area when giving a massage. The area is located near the vagina, and any stimuli are naturally tethered to her sexual organs. Use your hands or sensory play to tip the scales.

Inner Thighs

Any form of attention paid to the inner thighs of both women and men will get anybody in the mood for sex because they are so close to the genitalia. Sex is not just about the thrusting but the anticipation leading up to it. Make a submissive beg by paying close attention to this area with either the use of your hands, toys, paddles, or floggers.

Inner Wrist

The inside of a person's wrist is also considered an erogenous zone and does not commonly receive much attention. When out in public, be sure to stroke or tickle the inside of your partner's wrists. In the bedroom, intertwine your hands so that both yours and their wrists graze each other during sex.

For a more erotic approach, pay attention to this area by tracing the area with ice cubes or drip a few drops of candle wax to the area. The palm and fingertips are also sensitive areas of the hand.

Chapter 6: Light Play

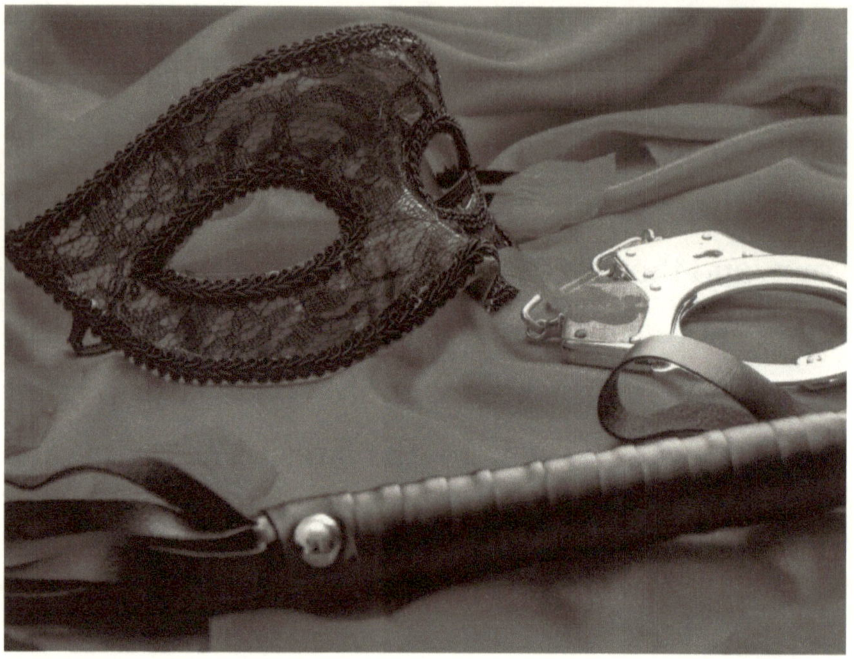

So you are into getting kinky, there is no problem with that. BDSM is not all scary, and there are many softer forms of play that you can bring into the bedroom in order to heat things up!

Household Items

Yes, you heard correctly. Before thinking of buying items online look in the cupboards at home for items that you can include in play, for example:

- **Clothing pegs** - Good for nipple stimulation, try the stomach area and inner thighs too, testing each other's limits. When removing the peg, it is important to add another stimulation like sucking or licking whichever body part to ease the sensation.
- **Spatula** - A great tool for spanking especially if the scene or moment is in the kitchen, just reach right over the counter!
- **Wooden spoon** - Another easily found and fantastic spanking tool.
- **Ruler** - An average household item that can spice up a spanking. Be careful as the rulers with a metal guide can leave marks.
- **Hairbrush** - The back end makes for a mild spanking tool, while the front bristle part works well for sensory play.
- **Scarf** - Makes for an ideal blindfold or bondage item. Always ensure that two fingers can be placed underneath the scarf, ensuring that circulation is not cut off.

- **Belt** - Could be used for flogging or in a softer manner as a restraint. Try wrapping the belt around your waist as a grip for the person to hold onto during sex, especially if they enter you from behind.
- **Gown cord** - A handy restraint tool.
- **Baby oil** - A useful addition perfect for sensual massages.
- **Foods** - Use some cream or chocolate sauce to ramp things up by licking them off each other. Please stay away from the fruit and vegetable drawer.

Though hanging up the laundry or wearing your favorite scarf might bring fits of giggles, it is worth trying.

Blindfold

Add a blindfold. By numbing one sense, all others are automatically heightened. The trick is to tempt and tease the individual, to keep them guessing as to what you will do next. The person without the blindfold is in power, and the blindfolded individual relinquishes power over to them. Feel free to tease your partner to the point of orgasm or use props such as a feather to tickle or dust over their bodies. Give them a spank, suck their nipples or ear lobes.

Hot or Cold Play

Candle wax is a household item that you can use when dabbling in sensory play. It sounds more daunting that what it is and isn't as painful as what you might imagine. Once again, it is a great way to test your limits and thresholds safely. Ensure you do your research as particular candles can burn differently, and you do not want to burn your partner. Be on the lookout for what is called "*safety candles*" readily available at local grocery and hardware stores. These are the ideal candles to use when contemplating wax play.

Alternatively, sex stores have massage candles, which burn at a lower heat and hold fragrant essential oils that make for the perfect overall body massage. You could add a dash of role-playing by one acting as a massage therapist and the other as a naive client.

On the other hand, the use of cold liquids such as ice water or ice-blocks is just as useful. You can either run the ice blocks up and down your partner's body or keep crushed ice in your mouth when kissing them or giving oral sex.

Biting

Biting is innocent enough and should not be done in a manner in which you maim your partner or draw blood. Once again start gently and progress to a harder bite. Some might find gazing down at a bite mark as a way to fantasize about that particular sexual encounter, whereas some might not appreciate marks left on their bodies.

Flogging and Spanking

Avoid a cane or a rod when first starting as it delivers a far more painful sensation than other items when undertaking *"impact play."* A wider surfaced paddle delivers a softer blow than a narrower one. A flogger is a leather whip with a woven handle and tails. It looks scary but isn't as painful. Whips come in a variety of styles, many are discreet and beautifully made, all delivering ranging feelings when used. Start slowly to find out each other's limits. These items can be purchased online via a multitude of sex stores. If whips do not appeal to you, you are welcome to make use of your hand or household items, as previously mentioned.

If you are receiving the flogging or spanking, why not suggest to your partner that you count the blows they intend to give. Your partner then has the opportunity to stagger the blows and their intensity, heightening your sexual arousal and excitement.

Name Calling

Name-calling does not need to be derogatory or shaming. Try using words such as *"sir," "madam,"* or "*master*." These names keep the fantasy and role-playing alive.

Talking Dirty

Talking dirty does not need to be aggressive or hurtful either. Rather it can be used as a way in which to guide your partner as to what you love, what you would like them to do, and what feels good. Talking dirty also builds up sexual tension and can increase orgasmic sensations. Go with what feels comfortable and in line with something you would say. Also, discuss this with your partner, what some might find kinky might be incredibly off-putting to the other.

Here are some phrases to help you on your way:

- "You are so sexy."
- "Do you like when I kiss you that way, what else do you like?"
- "See you later, lover."
- "I've been thinking about you all day."

- "You can't imagine the things I want to do to you."
- "Can I touch you?"
- "Do you like it when I..."
- "Looking at you makes me wet."
- "You make me so horny!"
- "I cannot stop thinking about last night/the other night."

These are all innocent enough sentences to use to aid you along and build your confidence when it comes to talking dirty. Obviously, you can add your own creative touch on them and become bolder in phrases.

Some stronger dirty talk that you can use:

- "I want to make you cum."
- "Cum for me."
- "I am your naughty girl, who is your naughty girl? Say it."
- "Fu-- me harder."
- "Scream my name."
- "I don't want you to stop, I want you inside me all night."

Tempt your partner even further by sending these in text messages, over social media or email, or when in a public space separately, or even together.

Hair Pulling

Hair pulling is a good way to start as it occurs quite organically while in the throes of passion. It can be a gentle tug or a harder pull. You determine the limits. The most pleasing effect is delivered if you pull the hair located at the nape of your partner's neck.

Run your fingers through your partner's hair towards the back of their head before getting a good grasp and giving it a pull, after which you gently release or hold on (less rigidly) for the ride. You can repeat this a few times during sex, foreplay or use when passionately kissing each other.

Fun Dress Play

Why not treat yourself to some lingerie, something unexpected that is comfortable and, of course, appealing. You do not need to scour the internet for full-body suits unless you really want to go full tilt.

Undress in front of them, wearing your new underwear. Send them a tempting photo of yourself when feeling frisky. Or next time you find yourself under the covers wear a pair of high-heeled stilettos or boots to liven things up.

Consider a pair of fishnet stockings, a leather or plaid mini skirt. Always alert your partner when you aren't wearing any underwear under a dress to get their mind racing.

Incorporate the following sensory items to tantalize and tease your partner or wear items made of:

- Feather
- Fur
- Lace
- Latex
- Leather
- Silk

Do not be afraid to use your nails, either.

Restraint

Invest in a pair of handcuffs or if you would like, purchase some rope from the hardware store with a softer feel so that neither grazes their limbs. As mentioned, a scarf can serve the same function. All need, want, and pleasure are placed in the dom's hands as there is no way a submissive can touch themselves or the dominant. Remember to keep the keys nearby. Restraint is the perfect way in which to practice orgasm control.

Sex Toys

There is a range of discreet sex toys on the market, all delivering a multitude of feelings and sensations. Invest in one good one that gets the job done and always keep a pack of extra batteries. The idea is to use it now and again and not for all sexual encounters with your partner. It can also be used as an aid to bring you near to orgasm and then for the partner to get you over the threshold. Pick out a toy that both of you can agree on something that you have chosen together.

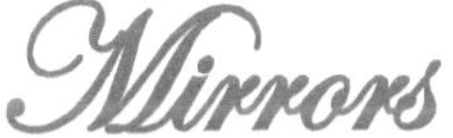 Mirrors

Many people become aroused at the thought of watching themselves having sex. Try having sex in front of a mirror. Role-playing and fantasies can be enhanced further by adding a mirror here and there.

Chapter 7: BDSM Games for the Bedroom

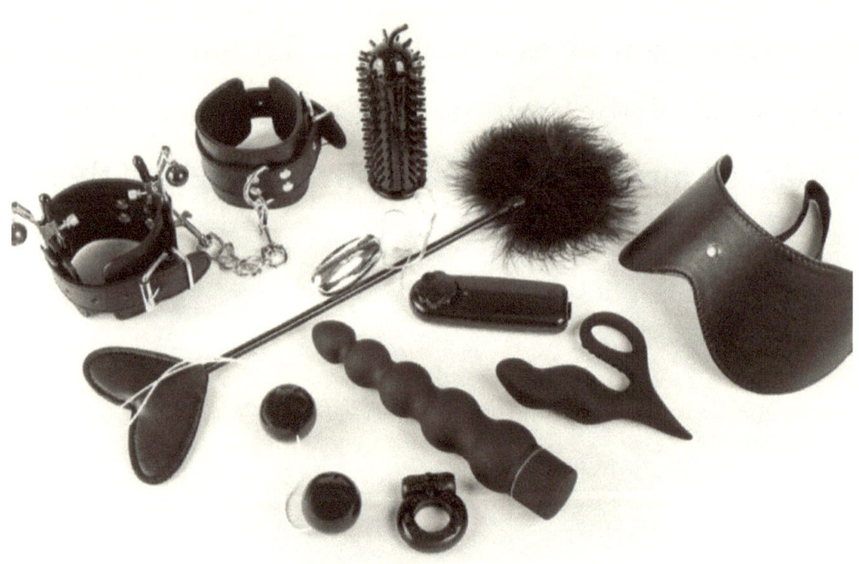

Sexually inspired games are a great way to add more heat to your sex life and build an even stronger level of intimacy with your partner. The games are not rules but guidelines and suggestions if you are unsure of how to go about them. All the games can be recreated or modified to suit your taste. Some of the games can include light play, costumes, and toys, which can clearly define either a submissive or dominant role or further emphasize a role-playing scenario.

Remember to always be able to laugh with your partner during these times, games need not be a serious matter and can also lead to just as pleasing sex without all the extras.

Beginner Games to Try

The games are simple to follow and, of course, easy well suited for the beginner who is tempted to discover more about BDSM and willing to bring more creativity to the bedroom.

A Roll of the Dice

Many online stores and sex shops have a variety of sexually inspired dice. These all hold various body parts, some indicating acts such as kissing or licking, and even sex positions. This a subtle way to mix things up in the bedroom. Toss the dice and follow the instructions, taking turns until you both come to orgasm.

As another option is that you can throw regular dice, depending on the number rolled dictates the number of minutes that your partner needs to go down on you.

BDSM Deck of Cards

Create your own deck of cards with BDSM inspired rewards and punishments. Throw in a few "*draw another card*" or "*double-ups*" to keep it interesting. Draw cards at random or during sex to keep things interesting. You can add new cards to the deck as you come up with new ideas in which to taunt and tease each other.

Orgasm Control

Orgasm control can result in the individual experiencing an ever stronger orgasm when given a chance. "*Edging*" is when you control the orgasm of a male specifically. The trick is to bring the person to the edge of orgasm and then stop all forms of stimulation so that they cannot finish. If you find yourself as the submissive, you place your orgasm in the hands of the dominant, which controls the scene and outcome thereof.

The dominant may use their hands, sex toys, or any other form of stimulation to bring you to the peak of orgasm and then stop. A suggestion is to keep doing this until you cannot contain it, the dominant will then take you to orgasm, be prepared for a mind-blowing bed shaking one!

Consider setting an alarm that goes off every minute or so, when this happens, you take turns stimulating each other; this is orgasm control at its best.

Gag Ball

Sex is no longer so much of a taboo as it once was, nor is erotic sex, and many stores sell a selection of gag balls, some of which are beautiful and less threatening. A dominant will use a gag ball to quieten a submissive. As a submissive, it adds a new range of feelings when not able to verbalize what you want.

Pretend that you are in a room full of people and that the aim of the dominant is to make you moan.

Collar

A collar defines the role as a submissive clearly and can be used in specific role-playing scenarios. A dominant might attach a leash to the collar to control the submissive during play.

Question Game

As a submissive, a dominant may ask you a set of questions. For every question you get right, you are rewarded. For every question that you get wrong, you are disciplined.

Rewards can be the following:

- One minute of oral sex
- Two minutes of stimulation with the use of a sex toy or hand
- Three minutes of penetrative sex

- Five minutes of passionate kissing

Discipline can include:

- Orgasm control

- No orgasm, only the dominant is allowed to

- Spanking

- 30 Seconds of nipple clamping

Playing in Public

Playing in public can consist of any acts that make you hot and bothered. It is important to keep in mind how and where you play so as not to break any laws. Public play involves not wearing any underwear, fondling, or even sex in public space such as a restaurant bathroom.

A dominant might also make use of a remote-controlled sex toy, for example, a wireless vibrating bullet. Your pleasure is in your partner's hands, and they determine the intensity and length of the vibrations.

You might also consider taping your sex to enjoy together on another occasion, or consider sending nude photos to each other in the middle of a work day.

Task Inspired Games

Tasks are often set out by the dominant for the submissive to complete and are commonplace in BDSM practice.

The point of the game is to set specific, goal-orientated activities for the submissive to try and do within a set time frame, such as making a cup of coffee or collecting something as simple as your handbag or mobile. If they complete the task in time, they are rewarded; if not, they are punished.

A dominant might choose even to distract the submissive, hampering their time to complete the task.

Love Swing

Invest in a door slam love swing that can easily be attached over the top of a closed door. It is bondage-inspired and perfect for couples tempted to try out new sex positions or a bit of BDSM. It is not bulky, nor is it difficult to assemble or disassemble. These swing sets are readily available online. They are adjustable and made to hold roughly 330 lb.

The swing set is great for role-playing, where a submissive takes on the role of somebody being held against their will. Place a mirror in front of the swing to get a birds-eye view of the action.

Role-Playing

It is easy to get stuck in a routine. That is why role-playing is an ideal way in which to bring variety into the bedroom. It also is another characteristic of the BDSM culture and a way in which to establish submissive and dominant roles.

Here are a few ideas to get you in the mood and to get your imagination going:

- Alien and abductee
- Strangers at a bar (Tip, try this at an actual bar or public space.)
- Professor and student

- Explorer and indigenous native
- Master and slave
- Bored housewife and pool boy (or repairman.)
- Sex worker and client
- Pirate and captive
- King and queen
- Kidnapper and the victim
- Photographer and model
- Daddy, daddy
- Fairytale characters
- Animals

The above are just a few examples of how you can bring fantasy elements into the bedroom. There are many other examples, and virtually no limitations when it comes to role-playing.

Remember to include extras to your role-playings such as costumes, bondage, blindfolds, and sex toys to further enhance the experience.

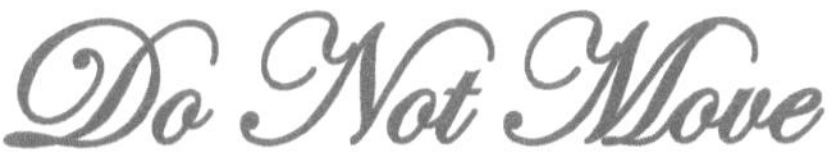

Do Not Move

In this game, the submissive is to remain still while the dominant pleases them. If the submissive moves, the dominant is allowed to discipline them in the manner in which they see fit. Once the punishment has been issued, the game may continue until the submissive experiences an orgasm.

Follow the Flogger

The submissive is required to keep in contact with the flogger, at all times. The dominant may set up obstacles to make this harder to achieve. If the submissive breaks contact with the flogger the dominant is allowed to discipline the submissive via spanking or with the use of the flogger. The game can continue like this until each other's anticipation becomes too great and ends in the bedroom.

Doll Play

The submissive may take on the role of a doll. Role-playing, make-up, and costumes go a long way to achieve this type of play. Just like a toy doll, the dominant may *"play"* with the doll in any way they would like.

Truth or Dare

When younger truth or dare was always an exciting game to play amongst friends. The aim of the game is simple, ask your partner a series of questions or dares based on sexual encounters or experiences.

For every time that you guess something correctly, your partner may move closer or act on a dare with sexual undertones. As a submissive tied up, this can equal great anticipation depending on the outcome of the dare or correctly or incorrectly answered questions.

Watch a Movie Together

The internet is the most useful tool that you have at your disposal in investigating the weird and rather wonderful world of BDSM. There are many porn sites available, all of which hold a multitude of categories depending on your preference. The idea for this game would be to find a BDSM inspired movie that you could watch together, copying the acts that you see.

Dom Worship

Why not try an evening solely catering to the needs and wishes of the dominant. Wear what they would like you to wear and act in a manner in which they would like. As the submissive, you offer up your pleasures to please them. The following evening the submissive may take on the role of the dominant.

Chapter 8: Games to Try for the More Adventurous

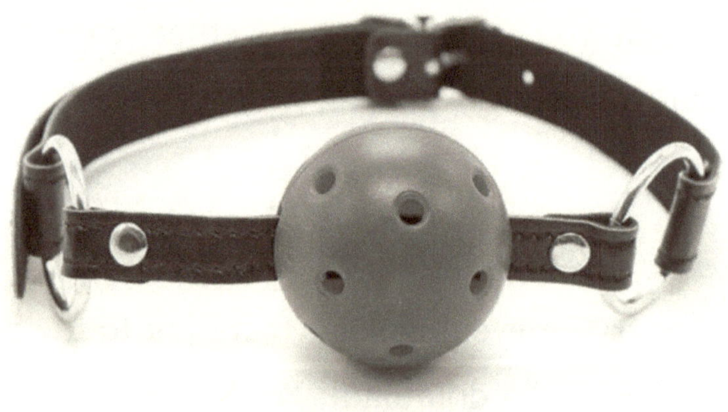

Perhaps you have already dabbled in a few of the games mentioned above or activities and are looking for more edgier, riskier forms of play. The three mentioned practices below guarantee to kick up your already kinkier types of play and definitely worth considering if you already own one or two general sex toys.

Cock Ring

A cock ring is a small, rather discreet sex toy that's aim is to keep the man going for longer. A male dominant or submissive may use one to delay orgasm. The ring is placed at the base of the penis. A silicone ring is best as it has no odor, it is durable and stretchy, plus it is considered comfortable, causing little to no friction. It is also small, so easy to store. Find them available online and in sex stores. These rings are great to get into a specific role and perfect for role-playing. A female dominant will enjoy using this on a male submissive as an effective teasing mechanism.

Penis Cage

As the name suggests, this is the perfect tool for a dominatrix. The penis-shaped, silicone cage is placed over a man's genitalia, prohibiting them from any sexual stimulation to that area of the body. They also come with a lock and keys, meaning the only release is up to the dominant. The dominatrix will then have free reign to seduce the submissive until they beg to be uncaged.

Anal Sex

Anal sex has a certain appeal to some people and does not have to be as daunting as it sounds. It can be pleasurable for both genders. Before you jump into it why not get used to the idea of anal sex by training your body to accept something going up the nether regions. Sex toys can be useful in this regard. Once you are willing to engage in anal sex, take it slow, use lube and consider trying it on a surface that is both comfortable and washable.

A submissive might find themselves on the receiving end of anal sex only if both parties consent to this. Do only what is comfortable. Like most BDSM practices, it is worth a try to figure out if it is something you want to continue.

"Pegging," the use of a strap on dildo to conduct anal sex might also be considered if a male partner would like to try anal sex or for those in a same-sex relationship.

Kama Sutra

Add a new erotic twist to your conventional sex position by studying the Kama Sutra. There are many dedicated books filled with kinky and sometimes rather strange, complex positions available online, or just search the internet for images based on this sexually enlightening read.

Why not undertake to try one to three new positions each time you find yourself in a sexual encounter. Randomly page to three sections within the book or cover your eyes and point to different positions, only discovering upon opening your eyes what they are.

For All to See

If your bedroom faces onto the street, why not consider opening the curtains next time you indulge in a bit of BDSM play. The public or neighbors will be provided with a free show. It makes for juicy conversation afterward as you talk about who saw, blushed, stared, or chose to ignore what they saw.

A bolder approach is to log in to online platforms, such as Periscope were live video feed is also available for all to see. You can then ask the public what you should do to your partner.

You may choose to sign out before things become explicit, or you may choose to keep the feed running for all to see your exploits. This game is good for those who find themselves in dominant and submissive roles; the dominant will follow the public's opinions within the submissive's limits, of course.

Chapter 9: Quickie Games

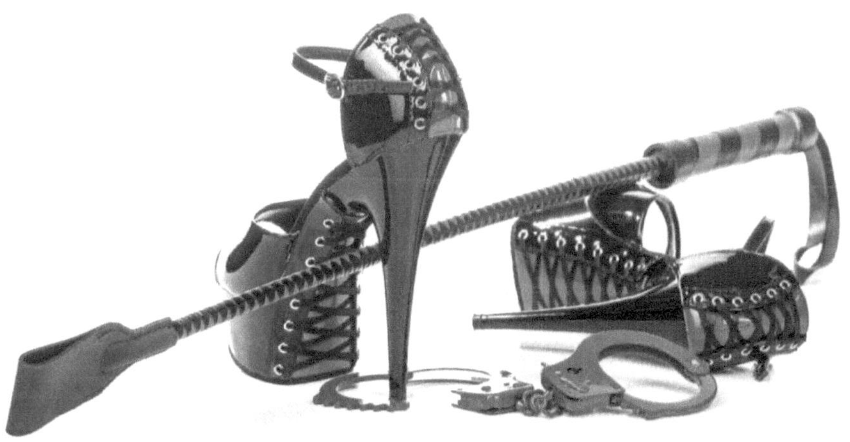

These sets of games are created to create some fun in the bedroom, and you are more than welcome to add your twist to them. Mix them up by adding costumes and toys.

Hide and Seek

Just as the game states, the submissive can hide anywhere in the house, and when the dominant finds them is allowed to issue a pleasure or punishment. Your partner can also seek you out and have sex where they find you.

Kinky Twister

Create your own twister inspired board game. The rules are simple, begin the game fully clothed; every time you cannot hold the pose or collapse, you remove an item of clothing. When both of you are naked, the game can continue, if the submissive stumbles the dominant may choose to stimulate them or discipline them.

Sexual Resolutions

Write down all the things that you would like to try sexually on separate pieces of paper. Encourage your partner to do the same. Place these resolutions, wishes, and wants into a jar. Every time you find yourself in the bedroom, choose to draw one of the pieces of paper and do what it says or if it is a bolder activity that needs planning to give yourself a week in which to follow through with it.

Sports

Watch a sports game, and each partner chooses an opposing team. Every Time your team scores a goal, you are allowed to dominate your partner and visa-versa. At the end of the game, the winner will take on the role as the dominant, and the loser will take on the role of the submissive.

Read a Book

Visit your local library or purchase an erotic novel online. Each partner may read a chapter out loud. Every time there is a sex scene mentioned, you can act this out on your partner, as described in the book.

Beat the Clock

Set a timer, say for five minutes. Either you can stimulate each other or yourself to see who comes to orgasm first before the alarm goes off. The winner takes on the role of the dominant, and the loser can take on the role of the submissive.

Erotic Jenga

Add an unconventional twist to a game of Jenga. Start the game off fully clothed; every time the tower collapses, the individual needs to remove an item of clothing. The game can continue when naked, and if the dominant causes the tower to come crashing down, they may please the submissive. If the submissive causes the tower to collapse, then the dominant may discipline them within their limits for 30 seconds to one minute.

Spin the Bottle

Both of you set ten items down in a circle, placing a bottle in the center. Items can include a blindfold, floggers, sex toys, whipped cream or a card with a suggestion written down on it. Each partner has a chance to spin the others bottle, whatever the bottle lands on they may apply or do to their partner.

Sensual Beer Pong

Lineup for an exciting night. Set the table out as you would for a game of beer pong, beer included. Start the game off fully clothed; every time your partner lands their ball in your cup, you are required to remove one item of clothing and down your drink.
The game can continue while naked and when the cups are empty. Every time the dominant lands a ball into the cup, they can punish the submissive. Every time the submissive lands their ball in the dominants cup, they are allowed to receive pleasure.

Sexy Scrabble

Leave the well-behaved, proper English words behind. Sexy scrabble takes on a whole new meaning when all you are allowed to do is spell out dirty, sexually-orientated words. For every point, remove an item of clothing. Continue while naked, for every point, the dominant get he or she may choose a punishment.

For every point, the submissive gets he or she may choose their pleasure. A dominant might decided, for example, if they get four points to either choose four various punishments, totally one minute or choose one punishment and do so for four minutes.

As you can no understand, BDSM covers almost all areas of sex. So if you have ever whipped out a scarf for a blindfold or spanked your partner with a belt then yes, you have engaged in BDSM. After this book you will know how acceptable it is to want to add acts and props to the bedroom to knock your partner's socks off and stimulate yourself like never before (all with consent of course).

It is important to know that if you choose to delve deeper into the world of BDSM that you conduct thorough research to keep all parties safe and revel in the pleasure. If you want to become good at something, you have to practice, and perfecting the art of BDSM is no different.

There is also a range of online chat rooms and forums where you can discuss your options with more experienced people in the BDSM community. Do not be nervous about approaching the topic with your partner nor seeking advice from others, even your friends. You may soon realize that many people have all sorts of tales to tell and kinks to share.

Each person is unique, and so are their sexual preferences and kinks. The idea is to share this passion go obtain gratification.

Start with a list of things that you would like to try, maybe try or never try; this can be the framework that you will use to begin your life-altering sex life. BDSM can be as gentle or as hard as you want it to be, that is the beauty of it and allows you to explore your sexual fantasies.

The art of placing your trust wholeheartedly in your partner's hands also holds a sense of danger and euphoria. This is what the acts and practices of BDSM offer those willing to lift the veil and find out how the other five million Americans are having sex.

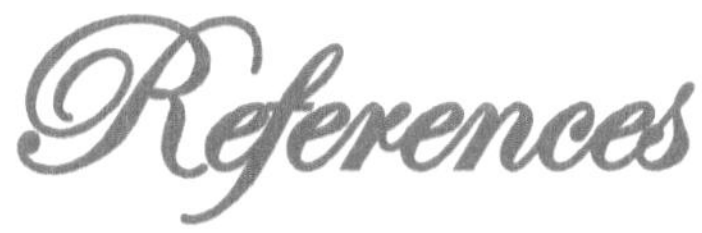

References

75 Filthy Sex Games That'll Make You Both Horny As Hell. (2018). Retrieved from https://thoughtcatalog.com/holly-riordan/2018/04/filthy-sex-games-thatll-make-you-both-horny-as-hell/

Aswell, S. (2019). Beginner's Guide to Kinky Sex: What Is It, Health Benefits, Rules. Retrieved from https://www.healthline.com/health/healthy-sex/kinky-sex-bdsm#the-rules-ofkink

Bacchus. (2019). Retrieved from https://simple.m.wikipedia.org/wiki/Bacchus

Bastion, N. (n.d.). 85 Sexy Dirty Talk Phrases Guaranteed to Make Him Ridiculously Turned On. Retrieved from https://www.vixendaily.com/love/dirty-talk-phrases-guaranteed-to-make-him-turned-on/5/

BDSM. (2019). Retrieved from https://en.wikipedia.org/wiki/BDSM

Breslaw, A., & Hsieh, C. (2019). Everything You Could Possibly Need to Know About Anal Sex. Retrieved from https://www.cosmopolitan.com/sex-love/advice/a6676/anal-sex-beginners-guide/

Frappier, I. (2019). 5 BDSM Games To Spice Up Your Sex Life Tonight - Top Story, Just the Tip. Retrieved from http://sexwithemily.com/5-bdsm-games/

Jameson, S. (2018). What Is BDSM: In-Depth Beginners Guide & Discover Why It's So Dam Enjoyable! Retrieved from https://badgirlsbible.com/what-is-bdsm

Jameson, S. (2018). 23 Kinky Sex Ideas: Very Freaky Tips To Spice Up Sex. Retrieved from https://badgirlsbible.com/kinky-sex-ideas

Jameson, S. (2018). Learn How To Be Submissive & Have Kinkier Sex. Retrieved from https://badgirlsbible.com/how-to-be-submissive

Kama Sutra. (2019). Retrieved from https://en.wikipedia.org/wiki/Kama_Sutra

LaFata, A. (2015). Erogenous Zones: 12 Unexpected Body Parts That Can Give You Pleasure. Retrieved from https://www.elitedaily.com/dating/unexpected-body-parts-pleasure/1115149

Lazarus, M. (2018). BDSM: How to be a Good Sub? Retrieved from https://beducated.com/mag/how-to-be-a-good-sub/

Matilda's - South Africa's Best Sex Toys & Adult Lingerie Store. (n.d.). Retrieved from https://www.matildas.co.za

McGowan, E. (2019). 13 Things To Try If You're New To BDSM. Retrieved from https://www.bustle.com/articles/133513-13-things-to-try-if-youre-new-to-bdsm

Megatron, S. (2019). How BDSM Is More Than Just a Sexual Practice. Retrieved from https://www.verywellmind.com/the-health-benefits-of-bdsm-2979720

Robinson, K. M. (2013). 10 Surprising Health Benefits of Sex. Retrieved from https://www.webmd.com/sex-relationships/guide/sex-and-health#

Sartore, M. (n.d.). Where Did BDSM Come From? Retrieved from https://www.ranker.com/list/discipline-and-dominance-origins/melissa-sartore

Soh, D. (2015). The truth about BDSM. Retrieved from https://www.independent.co.uk/life-style/love-sex/common-bdsm-myths-its-not-a-new-fad-its-not-violent-and-not-everyone-who-partakes-is-psychologically-a6702396.html

The Sanctuary of Artemis Orthia: History & Temple. (n.d.). Retrieved from https://study.com/academy/lesson/the-sanctuary-of-artemis-orthia-history-temple.html

Thomas, S. S. (2018). 8 BDSM Sex Tips to Try If You're a Total Beginner. Retrieved from https://www.allure.com/story/bondage-sex-tips-for-bdsm-beginners